The Super-Easy Keto Side Dishes Recipe Book

A Sensational Collection of Side Dishes Recipes for Your Keto Meals

Sebastian Booth

Table of contents

Warm Cauliflower Salad 5

Arugula & Roasted Pepper Salad 7

Smoked Salmon Salad 9

Greek Beef Meatball Salad 11

Caprese Salad Stacks with Anchovies...................14

Classic Greek Salad 16

Warm Mushroom & Pepper Salad 18

Cauliflower-Watercress Salad................................20

Shrimp Salad with Avocado....................................22

Green Salad with Feta & Blueberries....................24

Bacon & Gorgonzola Salad 26

Green Squash Salad 29

Chorizo & Tomato Salad with Olives.....................31

Tomato & Colby Cheese Salad................................33

Cranberry & Tempeh Broccoli Salad.....................35

Lettuce, Beet & Tofu Salad....................................37

Cream Soup with Avocado & Zucchini...................39

Chinese Tofu Soup..41

Summer Gazpacho with Cottage Cheese...............43

Fresh Avocado-Cucumber Soup 45

Zuppa Toscana with Kale 47

Awesome Chicken Enchilada Soup 49

Cauliflower Soup with Crispy Bacon 51

Reuben Soup..54

Mushroom Cream Soup with Herbs 56

Curried Shrimp & Green Bean Soup.......................................58

Hearty Vegetable Soup...60

Tomato Cream Soup with Basil 63

Spinach & Brussels Sprout Salad 65

Chicken Salad with Parmesan..67

Smoked Mackerel Lettuce Cups 69

Kale & Broccoli Slaw with Bacon & Parmesan 71

Turkey Bacon & Turnip Salad 73

Fiery Shrimp Cocktail Salad...75

Chicken, Avocado & Egg Bowls 78

Spinach Salad with Pancetta & Mustard.........................81

Mediterranean Artichoke Salad...83

Arugula & Watercress Turkey Salad 85

Spinach Salad with Goat Cheese & Nuts...........................88

Thai-Style Prawn Salad...90

Modern Greek Salad with Avocado 93

Seared Rump Steak Salad 95

Cheesy Beef Salad...98

Pickled Pepper Salad with Grilled Steak.........................101

Parma Ham & Egg Salad...103

Chicken Salad with Gorgonzola Cheese 105

Cheddar & Turkey Meatball Salad....................................108

Warm Cauliflower Salad

<u>Ingredients</u> for 4 servings

1 cup roasted bell peppers, chopped

2 tbsp celery leaves, chopped

10 oz cauliflower florets

1 red onion, sliced

¼ cup extra-virgin olive oil

1 tbsp wine vinegar

1 tsp yellow mustard

Salt and black pepper, to taste

½ cup black olives, chopped

½ cup cashew nuts

<u>Directions</u> and Total Time: approx. 15 minutes

Steam cauliflower in salted water in a pot over medium heat for 5 minutes; drain and transfer to a salad bowl. Add in roasted peppers, olives, and red onion.

In a small dish, combine salt, olive oil, mustard, black pepper, and vinegar. Sprinkle the mixture over the veggies. Top with cashew nuts and celery and serve.

Per serving: Cal 213; Fat 16g; Net Carbs 7.4g; Protein 5.2g

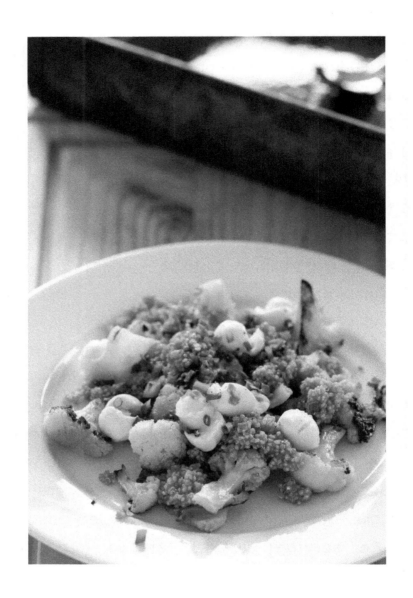

Arugula & Roasted Pepper Salad

<u>Ingredients</u> for 4 servings

2 lb red bell peppers, deseeded and cut into wedges

1/3 cup arugula

½ cup Kalamata olives, pitted

3 tbsp chopped walnuts

½ tsp Swerve sugar

2 tbsp olive oil

1 tbsp mint leaves

½ tbsp balsamic vinegar

¼ cup crumbled goat cheese

Toasted pine nuts for topping

Salt and black pepper to taste

<u>Directions</u> and Total Time: approx. 30 minutes

Preheat oven to 400 F. Pour bell peppers on a roasting pan; season with Swerve sugar and drizzle with half of the olive oil. Roast for 20 minutes or until slightly charred; set aside to cool.

Put arugula in a salad bowl and scatter with roasted bell peppers, olives, mint, walnuts, and drizzle with vinegar and olive oil. Season with salt and pepper. Toss and top with goat cheese and pine nuts.

Per serving: Cal 159; Net Carbs 4.3g; Fat 13g; Protein 3.3g

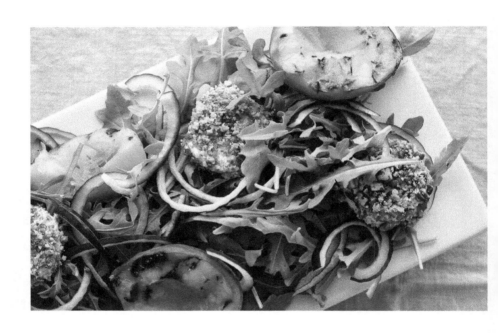

Smoked Salmon Salad

Ingredients for 2 servings

2 slices smoked salmon, chopped

1 tsp onion flakes

3 tbsp mayonnaise

½ Romaine lettuce, shredded

1 tbsp lime juice

1 tbsp extra virgin olive oil

Sea salt to taste

½ avocado, sliced

Directions and Total Time: approx. 10 minutes

Combine the salmon, mayonnaise, lime juice, olive oil, and salt in a bowl; mix to combine. On a salad platter, arrange the shredded lettuce and onion flakes. Spread the salmon mixture over and top with avocado slices.

Per serving: Cal 231; Fat 20g; Net Carbs 2.2g; Protein 8.5g

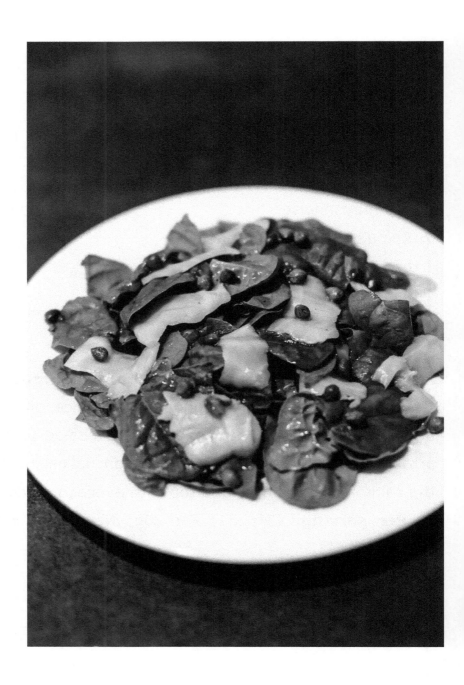

Greek Beef Meatball Salad

Ingredients for 4 servings

2 tbsp almond milk

1 lb ground beef

1 onion, grated

¼ cup pork rinds, crushed

1 egg, whisked

1 tbsp fresh parsley, chopped

Salt and black pepper, to taste

1 garlic clove, minced

1 tbsp fresh mint, chopped

½ tsp dried oregano

4 tbsp olive oil

1 cup cherry tomatoes, halved

1 Lebanese cucumber, sliced

1 cup butterhead lettuce, torn

1½ tbsp lemon juice

1 cup Greek yogurt

Directions and Total Time: approx. 20 minutes

In a bowl, mix the almond milk, ground beef, salt, onion, parsley, black pepper, egg, pork rinds, oregano, and garlic. Roll the mixture into balls. Warm half of the oil in a pan over medium heat and fry the meatballs for

8-10 minutes. Remove to a paper towel–lined plate to drain.

In a salad plate, combine lettuce, cherry tomatoes, and cucumber. Mix in the remaining oil, lemon juice, black pepper, and salt. Whisk the yogurt with mint and spread it over the salad; top with meatballs to serve.

Per serving: Cal 488; Fat 31g; Net Carbs 6.3g; Protein 42g

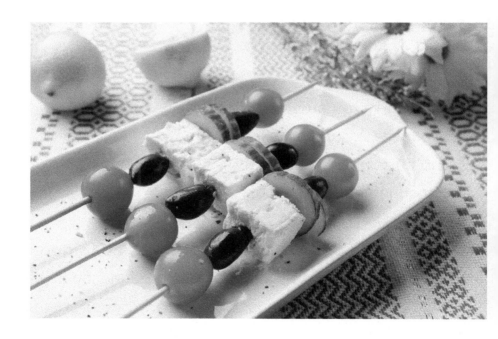

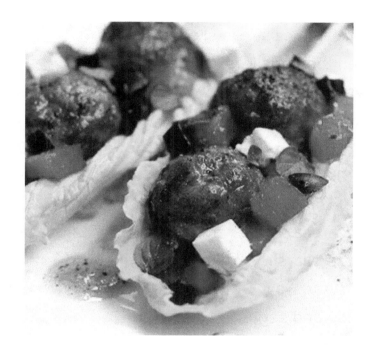

Caprese Salad Stacks with Anchovies

<u>Ingredients</u> for 4 servings

4 anchovy fillets in oil

12 fresh mozzarella slices

4 red tomato slices

4 yellow tomato slices

1 cup basil pesto

<u>Directions</u> and Total Time: approx. 10 minutes

Take a serving platter and alternately stack a tomato slice, a mozzarella slice, a yellow tomato slice, another mozzarella slice, a red tomato slice, and then a mozzarella slice on it. Repeat making 3 more stacks in the same way. Spoon pesto all over. Arrange anchovies on top and serve.

Per serving: Cal 182; Net Carbs 3.5g; Fat 6g; Protein 17g

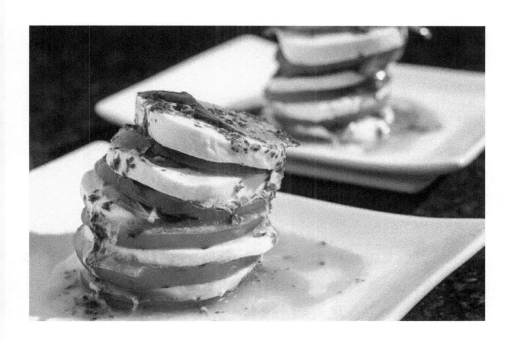

Classic Greek Salad

Ingredients for 2 servings

3 tbsp extra virgin olive oil

½ lemon, juiced

2 tomatoes, sliced

2 Persian cucumbers, diced

1 red bell pepper, sliced

1 small red onion, chopped

10 Kalamata olives

4 oz feta cheese, cubed

1 tsp parsley, chopped

Salt to taste

Directions and Total Time: approx. 10 minutes

Mix olive oil with lemon juice and salt in a bowl. In a salad bowl, combine tomatoes, cucumber, red onion, bell pepper, and parsley; toss with the dressing. Top with feta and olives. Serve.

Per serving: Cal 288; Fat 28g; Net Carbs 6.8g; Protein 10g

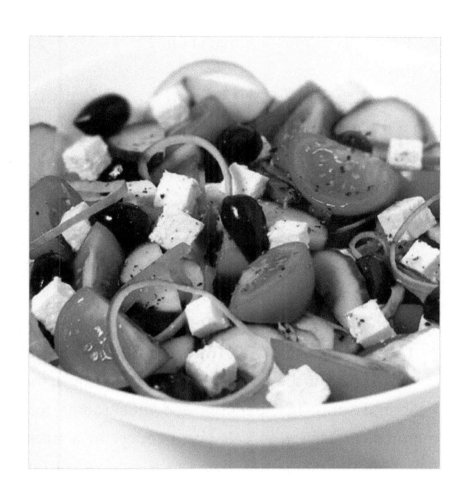

Warm Mushroom & Pepper Salad

Ingredients for 4 servings

1 cup mixed mushrooms, chopped

2 tbsp sesame oil

2 yellow bell peppers, sliced

1 garlic clove, minced

2 tbsp tamarind sauce

½ tsp hot sauce

1 tsp sugar-free maple syrup

½ tsp ginger paste

Chopped toasted pecans

Sesame seeds to garnish

Salt and black pepper to taste

Directions and Total Time: approx. 20 minutes

Warm half of the sesame oil in a skillet over medium heat and sauté bell peppers and mushrooms for 8-10 minutes. Season with salt and pepper. In a bowl, mix garlic, tamarind sauce, hot sauce, maple syrup, and ginger paste. Stir the mix into the vegetables and stir-fry for 2-3 minutes. Drizzle the salad with the remaining sesame oil and garnish with pecans and sesame seeds. Serve.

Per serving: Cal 291; Net Carbs 5.2g; Fat 27g; Protein 4.2g

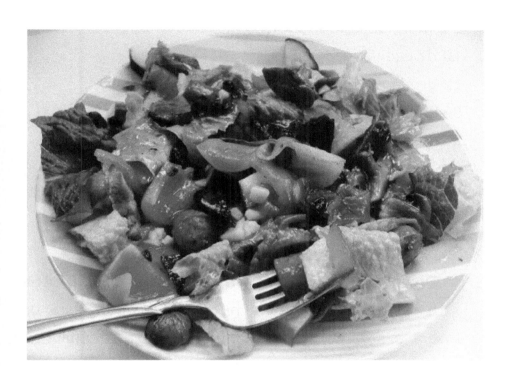

Cauliflower-Watercress Salad

Ingredients for 4 servings

2 tbsp sesame oil

1 lemon, zested and juiced

10 oz cauliflower florets

12 green olives, chopped

8 sun-dried tomatoes, drained

3 tbsp chopped scallions

A handful of toasted peanuts

3 tbsp chopped parsley

½ cup watercress

Salt and black pepper to taste

Directions and Total Time: approx. 15 minutes

In a pot over medium heat, bring water to a boil. Insert a steamer basket and pour in the cauliflower. Soften for 8 minutes. Transfer cauliflower to a salad bowl. Add in olives, tomatoes, scallions, lemon zest and juice, sesame oil, peanuts, parsley, and watercress. Season with salt and pepper and mix using a spoon. Serve.

Per serving: Cal 198; Net Carbs 6.4g; Fat 15g; Protein 6.6g

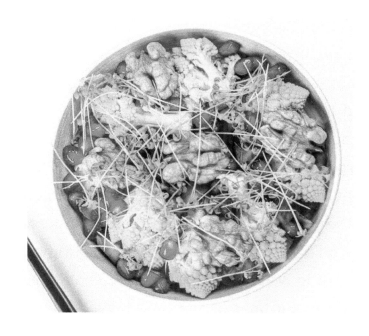

Shrimp Salad with Avocado

Ingredients for 4 servings

2 tomatoes, chopped

½ lb medium shrimp

3 tbsp olive oil

1 avocado, chopped

1 tbsp cilantro, chopped

1 lime, zested and juiced

1 head Iceberg lettuce, torn

Salt and black pepper to taste

Directions and Total Time: approx. 20 minutes

Heat 1 tbsp olive oil in a skillet over medium heat and cook the shrimp until opaque, 8-10 minutes. Place the lettuce on a serving plate and top with shrimp, tomatoes, and avocado. Whisk together the remaining olive oil, lime zest, juice, salt, and pepper in a bowl. Pour the dressing over the salad and sprinkle with cilantro to serve.

Per serving: Cal 229; Fat 18g; Net Carbs 4.2g; Protein 10g

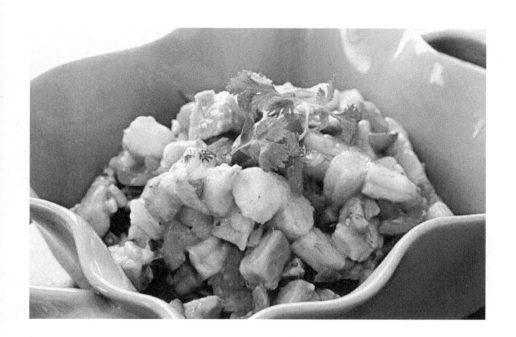

Green Salad with Feta & Blueberries

Ingredients for 4 servings

2 cups broccoli slaw

2 cups baby spinach

2 tbsp poppy seeds

1/3 cup sunflower seeds

1/3 cup blueberries

2/3 cup chopped feta cheese

1/3 cup chopped walnuts

2 tbsp olive oil

1 tbsp white wine vinegar

Salt and black pepper to taste

Directions and Total Time: approx. 10 minutes

In a bowl, whisk olive oil, vinegar, poppy seeds, salt, and pepper; set aside. In a salad bowl, combine the broccoli slaw, spinach, walnuts, sunflower seeds, blueberries, and feta cheese. Drizzle the dressing on top, toss, and serve.

Per serving: Cal 401; Net Carbs 4.9g; Fat 4g; Protein 9g

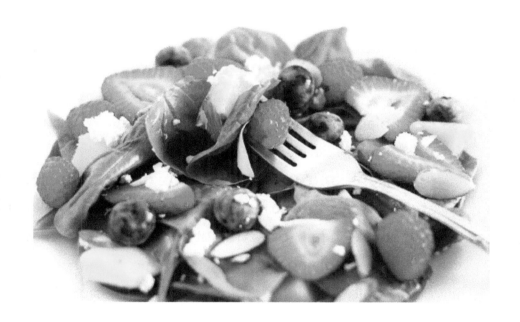

Bacon & Gorgonzola Salad

Ingredients for 4 servings

1 ½ cups gorgonzola cheese, crumbled

1 head lettuce, separated into leaves

4 oz bacon

1 tbsp white wine vinegar

3 tbsp extra virgin olive oil

Salt and black pepper to taste

2 tbsp pumpkin seeds

Directions and Total Time: approx. 15 minutes

Chop the bacon into small pieces and fry in a skillet over medium heat for 6 minutes, until browned and crispy. In a small bowl, whisk the white wine vinegar, olive oil, salt, and black pepper until dressing is well combined.

To assemble the salad, arrange the lettuce on a serving platter, top with the bacon and gorgonzola cheese. Drizzle the dressing over the salad, lightly toss, and top with pumpkin seeds to serve.

Per serving: Cal 339; Fat 32g; Net Carbs 2.9g; Protein 16g

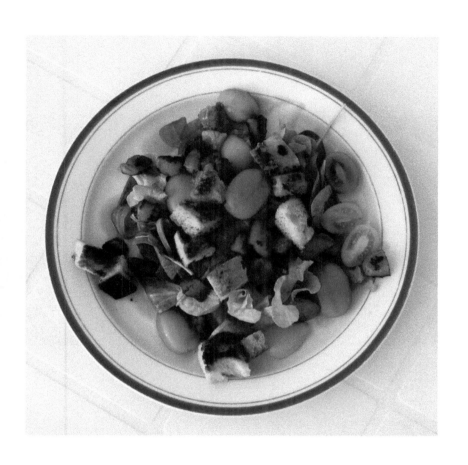

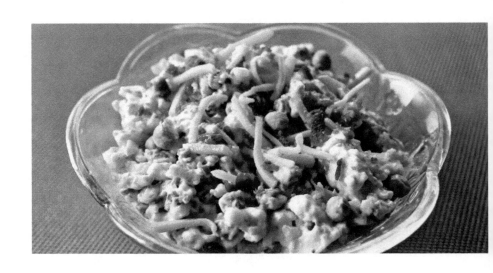

Green Squash Salad

Ingredients for 4 servings

2 tbsp butter

2 lb green squash, cubed

1 fennel bulb, sliced

2 oz chopped green onions

1 cup mayonnaise

2 tbsp chives, finely chopped

2 tbsp chopped dill

A pinch of mustard powder

Directions and Total Time: approx. 15 minutes

Place a pan over medium heat and melt butter. Fry squash until slightly softened, about 7 minutes; let cool. In a bowl, mix squash, fennel, green onions, mayonnaise, chives, and mustard powder. Garnish with dill.

Per serving: Cal 321; Net Carbs 3g; Fat 31g; Protein 4g

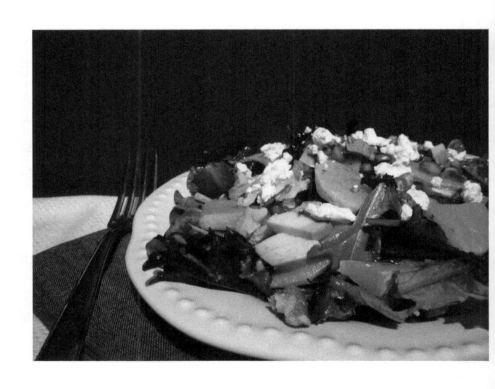

Chorizo & Tomato Salad with Olives

Ingredients for 4 servings

2 tbsp olive oil

4 chorizo sausages, chopped

2 ½ cups cherry tomatoes

2 tsp red wine vinegar

1 small red onion, chopped

2 tbsp chopped cilantro

8 sliced Kalamata olives

1 head Boston lettuce, shredded

Salt and black pepper to taste

Directions and Total Time: approx. 10 minutes

Warm 1 tbsp of olive oil in a skillet and fry chorizo until golden. Cut in half cherry tomatoes. In a salad bowl, whisk the remaining olive oil with vinegar, salt, and pepper. Add the lettuce, onion, tomatoes, cilantro, and chorizo and toss to coat. Garnish with olives to serve.

Per serving: Cal 141; Net Carbs 5.2g; Fat 9g; Protein 7g

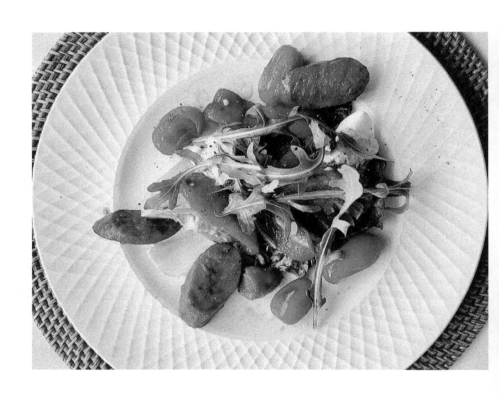

Tomato & Colby Cheese Salad

Ingredients for 2 servings

½ cucumber, sliced

2 tomatoes, sliced

½ yellow bell pepper, sliced

½ red onion, sliced thinly

½ cup colby cheese, cubed

10 green olives, pitted

½ tbsp red wine vinegar

4 tbsp olive oil

½ tsp dried oregano

Salt and black pepper to serve

Directions and Total Time: approx. 10 minutes

Place the bell pepper, tomatoes, cucumber, red onion, and colby cheese in a bowl. Drizzle red wine vinegar and olive oil all over and season with salt, pepper, and oregano; toss to coat. Top with olives and serve.

Per serving: Cal 578; Net Carbs 13g; Fat 51g; Protein 15g

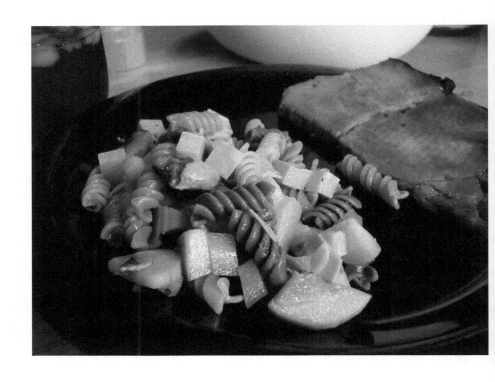

34

Cranberry & Tempeh Broccoli Salad

Ingredients for 4 servings

1 lb broccoli florets

¾ lb tempeh, cubed

2 tbsp butter

2 tbsp almonds

½ cup frozen cranberries

Salt and black pepper to taste

Directions and Total Time: approx. 15 minutes

In a deep skillet, melt butter over medium heat and fry tempeh cubes until brown on all sides. Add in broccoli and stir-fry for 6 minutes. Season with salt and pepper.

Turn the heat off. Stir in almonds and cranberries to warm through. Share the salad into bowls and serve.

Per serving: Cal 738; Net Carbs 7g; Fat 68g; Protein 12g

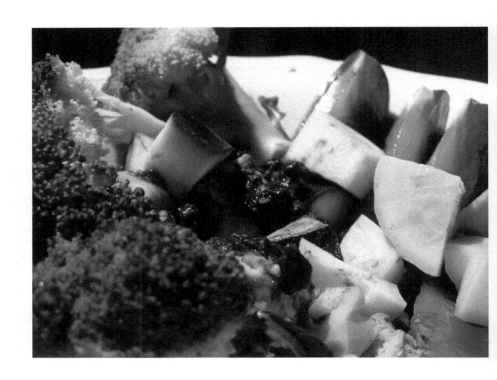

Lettuce, Beet & Tofu Salad

Ingredients for 4 servings

2 tbsp butter

2 oz tofu, cubed

8 oz red beets, washed

½ red onion, sliced

1 cup mayonnaise

1 small romaine lettuce, torn

2 tbsp freshly chopped chives

Salt and black pepper to taste

Directions and Total Time: approx. 55 minutes

Place the beets in a pot over medium heat, cover with salted water and bring to a boil for 40 minutes or until soft. Drain and allow cooling. Slip the skin off and slice the beets. Melt butter in a pan over medium heat and fry tofu until browned, 3-4 minutes. Remove to a plate.

In a salad bowl, mix beets, tofu, red onion, lettuce, salt, pepper, and mayonnaise. Garnish with chives and serve.

Per serving: Cal 415; Net Carbs 2g; Fat 40g; Protein 7g

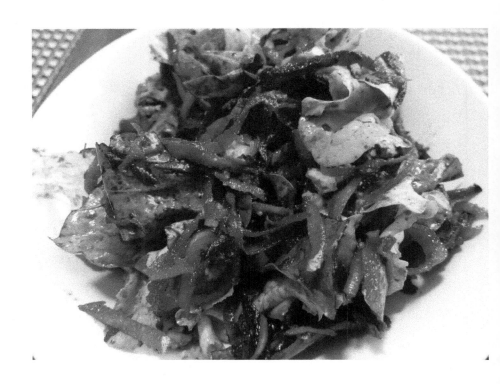

Cream Soup with Avocado & Zucchini

Ingredients for 4 servings

3 tsp vegetable oil

1 leek, chopped

1 rutabaga, sliced

3 cups zucchinis, chopped

1 avocado, chopped

Salt and black pepper to taste

4 cups vegetable broth

2 tbsp fresh mint, chopped

Directions and Total Time: approx. 40 minutes

Warm the vegetable oil in a pot over medium heat. Sauté the leek, zucchini, and rutabaga for 7-10 minutes. Season with pepper and salt. Pour in broth and bring to a boil. Lower the heat and simmer for 20 minutes. Lift from the heat. In batches, add the soup and avocado to a blender. Blend until creamy and smooth. Top with mint and serve.

Per serving: Cal 378; Fat 24.5g; Net Carbs 9.3g; Protein 8g

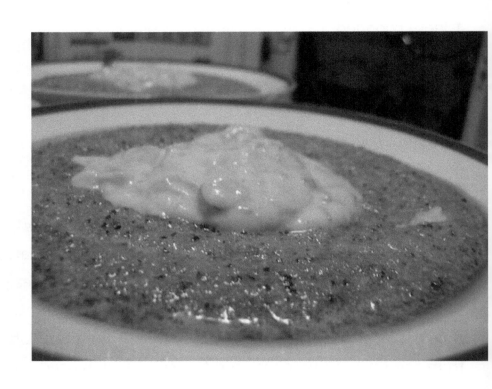

Chinese Tofu Soup

Ingredients for 2 servings

2 cups chicken stock

1 tbsp soy sauce, sugar-free

2 spring onions, sliced

1 tsp sesame oil, softened

2 eggs, beaten

1-inch piece ginger, grated

Salt and black pepper to taste

½ lb extra-firm tofu, cubed

1 tbsp fresh cilantro, chopped

Directions and Total Time: approx. 15 minutes

Boil in a pan over medium heat, soy sauce, chicken stock and sesame oil. Place in eggs as you whisk to incorporate thoroughly. Change heat to low and add salt, spring onions, black pepper and ginger; cook for 5 minutes. Place in tofu and simmer for 1 to 2 minutes. Divide into soup bowls and serve sprinkled with fresh cilantro.

Per serving: Cal 163; Fat 10g; Net Carbs 2.4g; Protein 14g

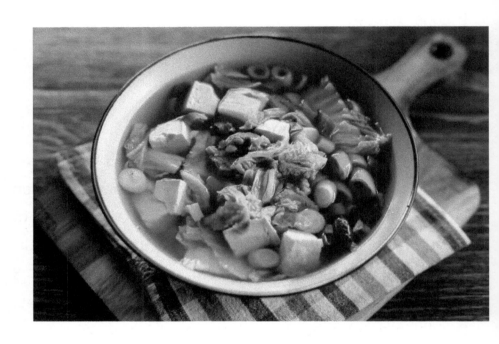

Summer Gazpacho with Cottage Cheese

Ingredients for 4 servings

1 green pepper, roasted

1 red pepper, roasted

1 avocado, flesh scoped out

1 garlic clove

1 spring onion, chopped

1 cucumber, chopped

½ cup olive oil

1 tbsp lemon juice

2 tomatoes, chopped

4 oz cottage cheese, crumbled

1 small red onion, chopped

1 tbsp apple cider vinegar

Salt to taste

Directions and Total Time: approx. 15 min + cooling time

In a blender, put the peppers, tomatoes, avocado, red onion, garlic, lemon juice, olive oil, vinegar, half of the cucumber, 1 cup of water, and cottage cheese. Blitz until your desired consistency is reached; adjust the seasoning.Transfer the mixture to a pot. Cover and chill in the fridge for at least 2 hours. Serve the soup topped with the remaining cucumber, spring onion, and an extra drizzle of olive oil.

Per serving: Cal 373; Fat 34g; Net Carbs 7.1g; Protein 5.8g

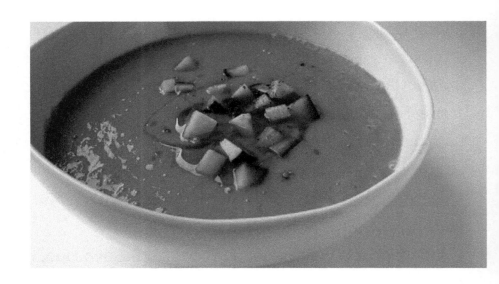

Fresh Avocado-Cucumber Soup

Ingredients for 4 servings

3 tbsp olive oil

1 small onion, chopped

4 large cucumbers, chopped

1 avocado, peeled and pitted

Salt and black pepper to taste

1 ½ cups water

½ cup Greek yogurt

1 tbsp cilantro, chopped

2 limes, juiced

1 garlic clove, minced

2 tomatoes, chopped

1 chopped avocado

Directions and Total Time: approx. 10 min + cooling time

Pour all the ingredients, except for the tomatoes and avocado, into the food processor. Puree for 2 minutes or until smooth. Pour the mixture into a bowl. Cover and refrigerate for 2 hours. Top with avocado and tomatoes.

Per serving: Cal 343; Fat 26g; Net Carbs 5.3g; Protein 10g

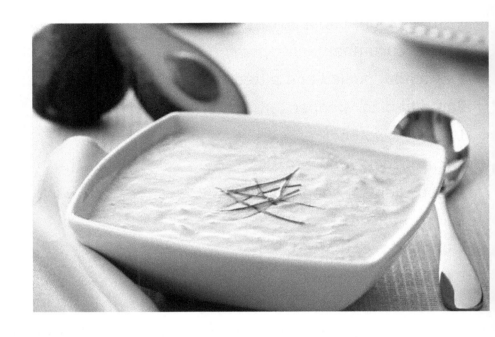

Zuppa Toscana with Kale

Ingredients for 4 servings

2 cups chicken broth

1 tbsp olive oil

¼ cup heavy cream

1 cup kale

3 oz pancetta, chopped

1 parsnip, chopped

1 garlic clove, minced

Salt and black pepper, to taste

¼ tsp red pepper flakes

½ onion, chopped

1 lb hot Italian sausage, sliced

2 tbsp Parmesan, grated

Directions and Total Time: approx. 40 minutes

Warm the olive oil in a pan over medium heat. Stir-fry the garlic, onion, pancetta, and sausage for 5 minutes. Pour in chicken broth and parsnip and simmer for 15-20 minutes. Stir in the remaining ingredients, except for the Parmesan cheese, and cook for about 5 minutes. Serve topped with Parmesan cheese.

Per serving: Cal 543; Fat 45g; Net Carbs 5.6g; Protein 24g

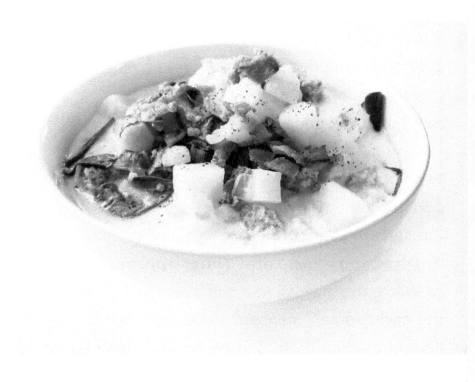

Awesome Chicken Enchilada Soup

<u>Ingredients</u> for 4 servings

½ lb boneless, skinless chicken thighs

2 tbsp coconut oil

¾ cup red enchilada sauce

1 onion, chopped

3 oz canned diced green chilis

1 avocado, sliced

1 cup cheddar, shredded

1 pickled jalapeño, chopped

½ cup sour cream

1 tomato, diced

<u>Directions</u> and Total Time: approx. 35 minutes

Put a large pan over medium heat. Add coconut oil and warm. Place in the chicken and cook until browned on the outside. Stir in onion, jalapeño, and green chilis and cook for 2 minutes. Pour in 4 cups of water and enchilada sauce. Allow simmering for 20 minutes until the chicken is cooked through. Spoon the soup on a serving bowl and top with the cheese, sour cream, tomato, and avocado.

Per serving: Cal 643; Fat 44g; Net Carbs 9.7g; Protein 48g

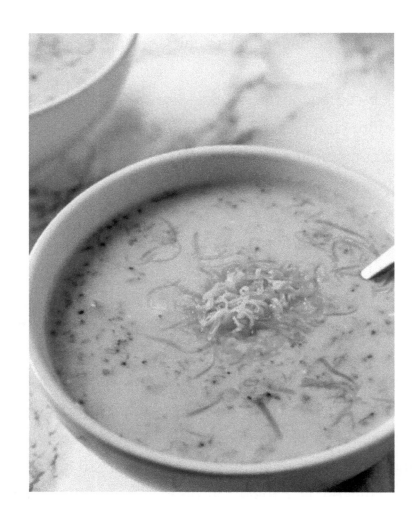

Cauliflower Soup with Crispy Bacon

Ingredients for 4 servings

2 tbsp olive oil

1 onion, chopped

¼ celery root, grated

10 oz cauliflower florets

Salt and black pepper to taste

1 cup almond milk

1 cup white cheddar, shredded

2 oz bacon, cut into strips

Directions and Total Time: approx. 25 minutes

Heat a skillet over medium heat and fry the bacon for 5 minutes until crispy; set aside on a paper towel–lined plate. In the same skillet, add warm the olive oil and sauté the onion for 3 minutes until fragrant. Include the cauliflower florets and celery root and sauté for 3 minutes until slightly softened. Add 3 cups of water and season with salt and pepper. Bring to a boil, and then reduce the heat to low. Cover and cook for 10 minutes.

Puree the soup with an immersion blender until the ingredients are evenly combined and stir in the almond milk and cheese until it melts. Adjust taste with salt and black pepper. Top with crispy bacon and serve hot.

Per serving: Cal 323; Fat 27g; Net Carbs 7.6g; Protein 23g

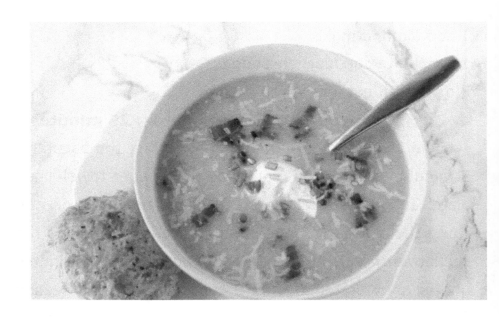

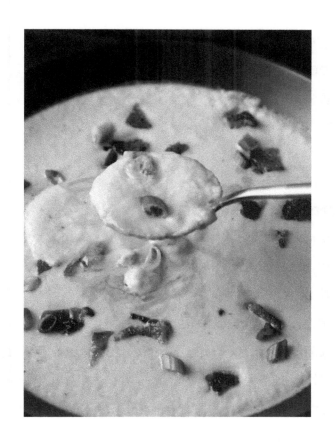

Reuben Soup

Ingredients for 4 servings

1 parsnip, chopped

1 onion, diced

3 cups beef stock

1 celery stalk, diced

1 garlic clove, minced

1 cup heavy cream

½ cup sauerkraut, shredded

½ lb corned beef, chopped

2 tbsp lard

½ cup mozzarella, shredded

Salt and black pepper, to taste

Chopped chives for garnish

Directions and Total Time: approx. 30 minutes

Melt the lard in a large pot. Add parsnip, onion, garlic, and celery and fry for 3 minutes until tender.

Pour the beef stock over and stir in sauerkraut, salt, and black pepper. Bring to a boil. Reduce the heat to low, and add the corned beef. Cook for about 15 minutes, adjust the seasoning. Stir in heavy cream and cheese and cook for 1 minute. Garnish with chives to serve.

Per serving: Cal 463; Fat 41g; Net Carbs 5.8g; Protein 21g

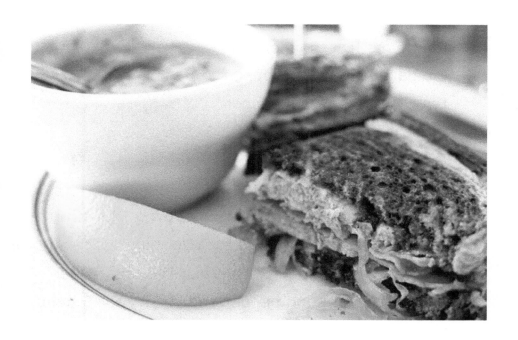

Mushroom Cream Soup with Herbs

Ingredients for 4 servings

12 oz white mushrooms, chopped

1 onion, chopped

½ cup heavy cream

¼ cup butter

1 tsp thyme leaves, chopped

1 tsp parsley leaves, chopped

1 tsp cilantro leaves, chopped

2 garlic cloves, minced

4 cups vegetable broth

Salt and black pepper to taste

Directions and Total Time: approx. 25 minutes

Melt the butter in a large pot over high heat and cook the onion and garlic for 3 minutes until tender. Add mushrooms, salt, and pepper and stir-fry for 5 minutes. Pour in the broth and bring to a boil. Reduce heat and simmer for 10 minutes. Puree soup with a hand blender until smooth. Stir in heavy cream. Garnish with herbs.

Per serving: Cal 292; Fat 25.2g; Net Carbs 3.4g; Protein 8g

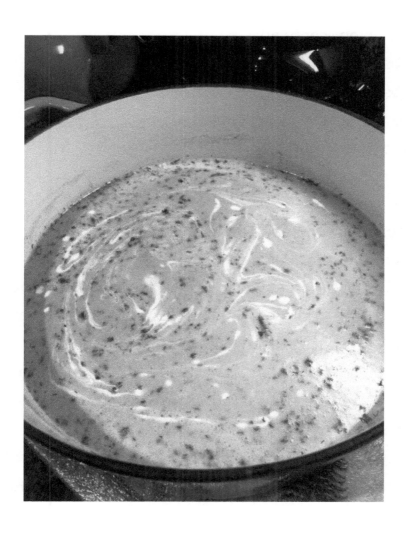

Curried Shrimp & Green Bean Soup

Ingredients for 4 servings

1 onion, chopped

2 tbsp red curry paste

2 tbsp butter

1 lb jumbo shrimp, deveined

2 tsp ginger-garlic puree

1 cup coconut milk

Salt and chili pepper to taste

1 bunch green beans, halved

1 tbsp cilantro, chopped

Directions and Total Time: approx. 20 minutes

Add the shrimp to melted butter in a saucepan over medium heat, season with salt and pepper, and cook until they are opaque, 2-3 minutes. Remove to a plate. Add in the ginger-garlic puree, onion, and red curry paste and sauté for 2 minutes until fragrant.

Stir in the coconut milk and add the shrimp, salt, chili pepper, and green beans. Cook for 4 minutes. Reduce the heat to a simmer and cook an additional 3 minutes, occasionally stirring. Adjust the taste with salt. Fetch the soup into serving bowls and sprinkle with cilantro.

Per serving: Cal 351; Fat 32g; Net Carbs 3.2g; Protein 7.7g

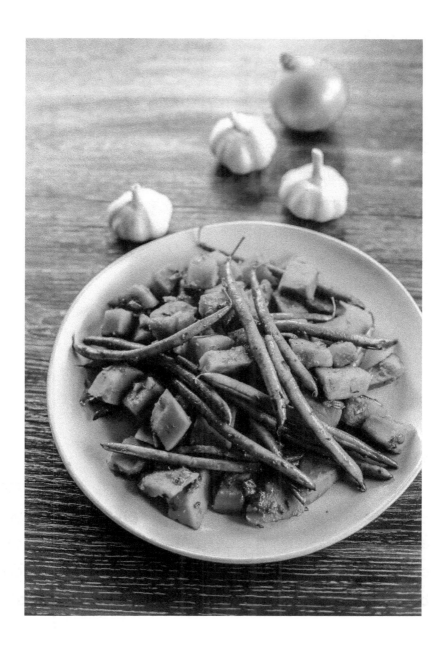

Hearty Vegetable Soup

<u>Ingredients</u> for 4 servings

2 tsp olive oil

1 onion, chopped

1 garlic clove, minced

½ celery stalk, chopped

1 cup mushrooms, sliced

½ head broccoli, chopped

½ carrot, sliced

1 cup spinach, torn into pieces

Salt and black pepper, to taste

2 thyme sprigs, chopped

½ tsp dried rosemary

3 cups vegetable stock

1 tomato, chopped

½ cup almond milk

<u>Directions</u> and Total Time: approx. 35 minutes

Heat olive oil in a saucepan. Add onion, celery, garlic, and carrot and sauté until translucent, stirring occasionally, about 5 minutes. Place in the mushrooms, broccoli, salt, rosemary, tomatoes, pepper, thyme, and vegetable stock. Simmer the mixture for 15 minutes while the lid is slightly open. Stir in almond milk and spinach and cook for 5 more minutes. Serve.

Per serving: Cal 167; Fat 6.2g; Net Carbs 7.9g; Protein 3.2g

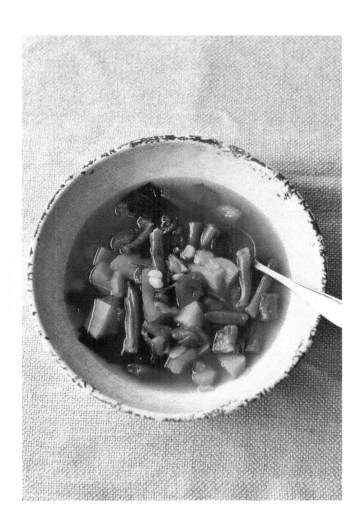

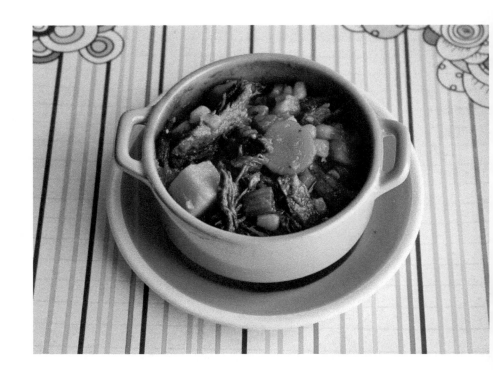

Tomato Cream Soup with Basil

Ingredients for 4 servings

1 carrot, chopped

2 tbsp olive oil

1 onion, diced

1 garlic clove, minced

¼ cup raw cashew nuts, diced

14 oz canned tomatoes

1 tsp fresh basil leaves

Salt and black pepper to taste

1 cup crème fraîche

Directions and Total Time: approx. 25 minutes

Warm olive oil in a pot over medium heat and sauté the onion, carrot, and garlic for 4 minutes until softened. Stir in the tomatoes and 2 cups of water and season with salt and black pepper. Cover and bring to simmer for 10 minutes until thoroughly cooked. Puree the ingredients with an immersion blender. Adjust to taste and stir in the crème fraîche and cashew nuts. Serve topped with basil.

Per serving: Cal 253; Fat 23g; Net Carbs 6g; Protein 4g

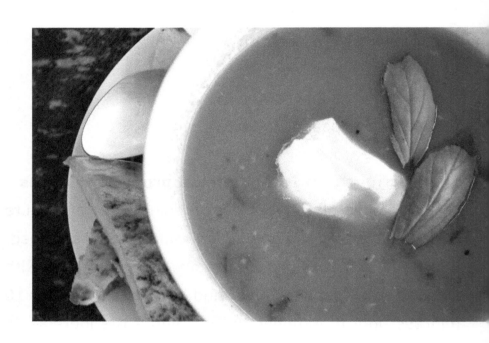

Spinach & Brussels Sprout Salad

<u>Ingredients</u> for 2 servings

1 lb Brussels sprouts, halved

2 tbsp olive oil

Salt and black pepper to taste

1 tbsp balsamic vinegar

2 tbsp extra virgin olive oil

1 cup baby spinach

1 tbsp Dijon mustard

½ cup hazelnuts

<u>Directions</u> and Total Time: approx. 35 minutes

Preheat oven to 400 F. Drizzle the Brussels sprouts with olive oil, sprinkle with salt and pepper, and spread on a baking sheet. Bake until tender, 20 minutes, tossing often.

In a dry pan over medium heat, toast the hazelnuts for 2 minutes, cool, and then chop into small pieces. Transfer the Brussels sprouts to a salad bowl and add the baby spinach. Mix until well combined. In a small bowl, combine vinegar, mustard, and olive oil. Drizzle the dressing over the salad and top with hazelnuts to serve.

Per serving: Cal 511; Fat 43g; Net Carbs 9.6g; Protein 14g

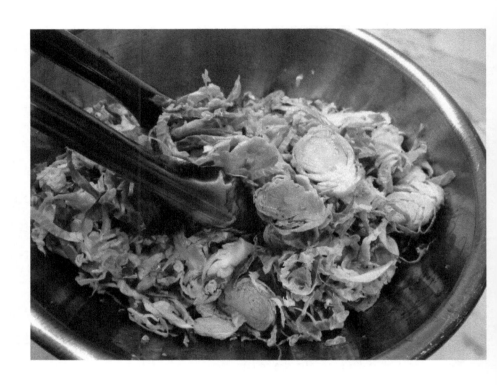

Chicken Salad with Parmesan

Ingredients for 2 servings

½ lb chicken breasts, sliced

¼ cup lemon juice

2 garlic cloves, minced

2 tbsp olive oil

1 romaine lettuce, shredded

3 Parmesan crisps

2 tbsp Parmesan, grated

Dressing

2 tbsp extra virgin olive oil

1 tbsp lemon juice

Salt and black pepper to taste

Directions and Total Time: approx. 30 min + chilling time

In a Ziploc bag, put the chicken, lemon juice, oil, and garlic. Seal the bag, shake to combine, and refrigerate for 1 hour.

Preheat the grill to medium heat and grill the chicken for about 2-3 minutes per side. Combine the dressing ingredients in a small bowl and mix well. On a serving platter, arrange the lettuce and Parmesan crisps. Scatter the dressing over and toss to coat. Top with the chicken and Parmesan cheese to serve.

Per serving: Cal 529; Fat 36g; Net Carbs 4.3g; Protein 34g

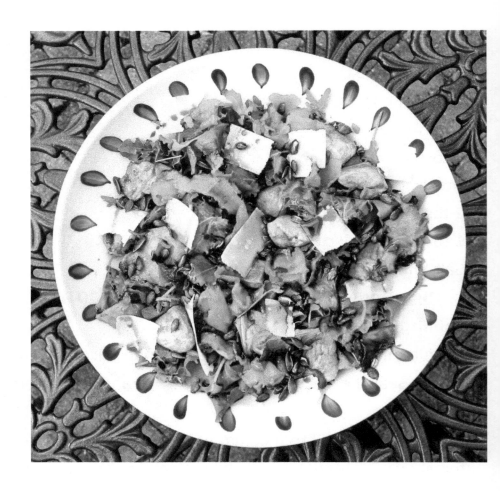

Smoked Mackerel Lettuce Cups

Ingredients for 2 servings

½ head Iceberg lettuce, firm leaves removed for cups

4 oz smoked mackerel, flaked

Salt and black pepper to taste

2 eggs

1 tomato, seeded, chopped

2 tbsp mayonnaise

¼ red onion, sliced

1 tsp lemon juice

1 tbsp chives, chopped

Directions and Total Time: approx. 20 minutes

Boil the eggs in a small pot with salted water for 10 minutes. Then, run the eggs in cold water, peel, and chop into small pieces. Transfer them to a salad bowl. Add in the smoked mackerel, red onion, and tomato and mix evenly with a spoon. Mix the mayonnaise, lemon juice, salt, and pepper in a small bowl and stir to combine. Lay two lettuce leaves each as cups and divide the salad mixture between them. Sprinkle with chives and serve.

Per serving: Cal 314; Fat 25g; Net Carbs 3g; Protein 16g

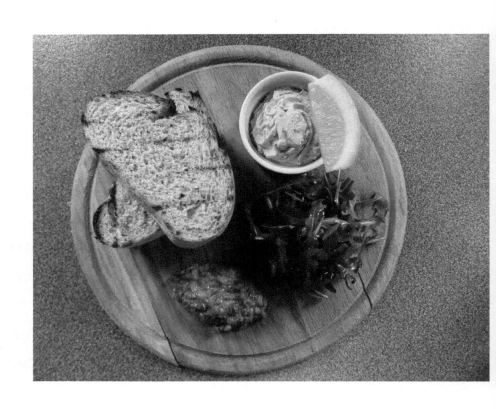

Kale & Broccoli Slaw with Bacon & Parmesan

Ingredients for 2 servings

2 tbsp olive oil

1 cup broccoli slaw

1 cup kale slaw

2 slices bacon, chopped

2 tbsp Parmesan, grated

1 tsp celery seeds

1 ½ tbsp apple cider vinegar

Salt and black pepper, to taste

Directions and Total Time: approx. 10 minutes

Fry the bacon in a skillet over medium heat until crispy, about 5 minutes. Set aside to cool. In a salad bowl, whisk the olive oil, vinegar, salt, and pepper. Add in the broccoli, kale, and celery seeds and mix to combine well. Sprinkle with bacon and Parmesan and serve.

Per serving: Cal 305; Fat 29g; Net Carbs 3.7g; Protein 7.3g

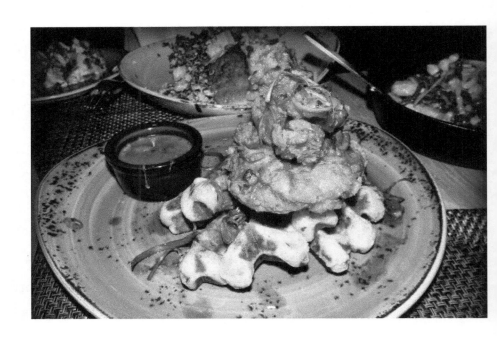

Turkey Bacon & Turnip Salad

Ingredients for 4 servings

2 turnips, cut into wedges

2 tsp olive oil

1/3 cup black olives, sliced

1 cup baby spinach

6 radishes, sliced

3 oz turkey bacon, sliced

4 tbsp buttermilk

2 tsp mustard seeds

1 tsp Dijon mustard

1 tbsp red wine vinegar

Salt and black pepper to taste

1 tbsp chives, chopped

Directions and Total Time: approx. 40 minutes

Fry the turkey bacon in a skillet over medium heat until crispy, about 5 minutes. Set aside, then crumble it.

Line a baking sheet with parchment paper, toss the turnips with black pepper, drizzle with the olive oil, and bake in the oven for 25 minutes at 390 F, turning halfway through. Let cool. Spread the baby spinach at the bottom of a salad platter and top with the radishes, bacon, and turnips. Mix the buttermilk, mustard seeds, mustard, vinegar, and salt. Pour the dressing over the salad, stir well and scatter with the chives and olives to serve.

Per serving: Cal 95; Fat 5g; Net Carbs 3.4g; Protein 6g

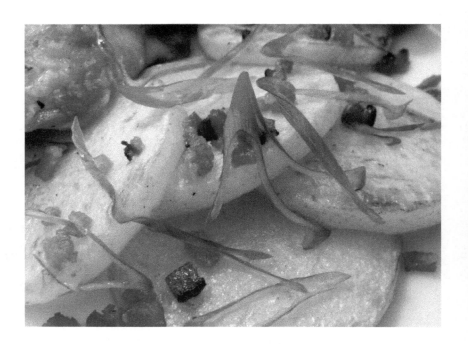

Fiery Shrimp Cocktail Salad

<u>Ingredients</u> for 4 servings

2 tbsp olive oil

½ head Romaine lettuce, torn

1 cucumber, cut into ribbons

½ lb shrimp, deveined

1 cup arugula

½ cup mayonnaise

2 tbsp Cholula hot sauce

½ tsp Worcestershire sauce

Salt and chili pepper to season

1 tbsp lemon juice

1 lemon, cut into wedges

4 dill weed

<u>Directions</u> and Total Time: approx. 15 min + cooling time

Season the shrimp with salt and chili pepper. Warm the olive oil over medium heat and fry the shrimp for 3 minutes on each side until pink and opaque. Set aside to cool. Place the mayonnaise, lemon juice, hot sauce, and Worcestershire sauce and mix until smooth and creamy in a bowl. Divide the lettuce and cucumber between 4 glass bowls. Top with shrimp and drizzle the hot dressing over. Scatter arugula on top and decorate with lemon wedges and dill to serve.

Per serving: Cal 201; Fat 11g; Net Carbs 3.9g; Protein 14g

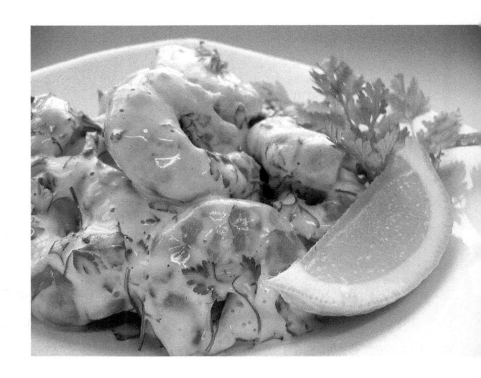

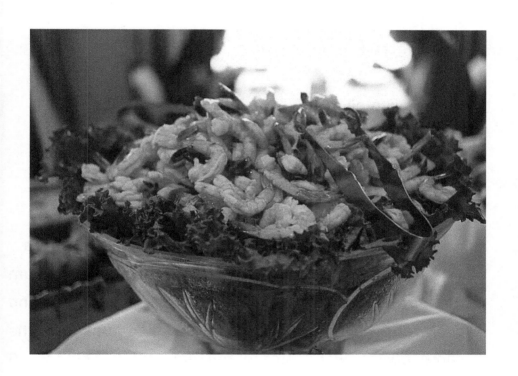

Chicken, Avocado & Egg Bowls

Ingredients for 2 servings

1 chicken breast, cubed

1 tbsp avocado oil

2 eggs

2 cups green beans

1 avocado, sliced

2 tbsp olive oil

2 tbsp lemon juice

1 tsp Dijon mustard

1 tbsp mint, chopped

Salt and black pepper to taste

Directions and Total Time: approx. 25 minutes

Blanch the green beans in salted water over medium heat for 4-5 minutes until the beans are bright green and crisp-tender. Refresh in cold water and drain. In the same boiling water, place the eggs and cook for 10 minutes. Remove to an ice bath to cool. Then, peel and slice them.

Warm the avocado oil in a pan over medium heat. Cook the chicken for about 4 minutes. Divide the green beans between two salad bowls. Top with chicken, eggs, and avocado slices. In another bowl, whisk together the lemon juice, olive oil, mustard, salt, and pepper, and drizzle over the salad. Top with fresh mint and serve.

Per serving: Cal 612; Fat 48g; Net Carbs 6.9g; Protein 27g

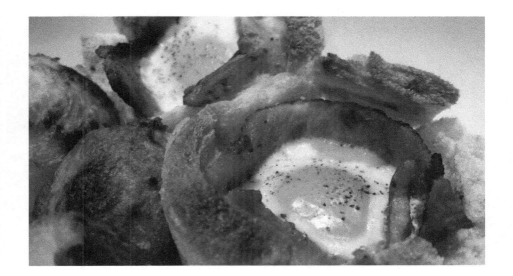

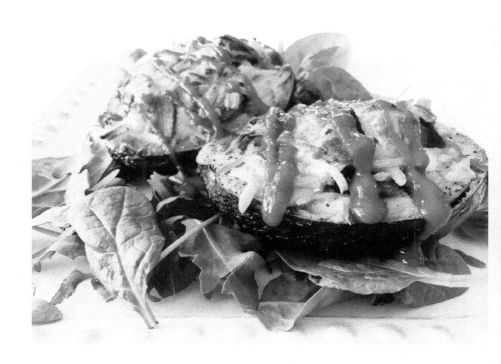

Spinach Salad with Pancetta & Mustard

<u>Ingredients</u> for 2 servings

1 cup spinach

1 large avocado, sliced

1 spring onion, sliced

2 pancetta slices

½ lettuce head, shredded

1 hard-boiled egg, chopped

Vinaigrette

Salt to taste

¼ tsp garlic powder

3 tbsp olive oil

1 tsp Dijon mustard

1 tbsp white wine vinegar

<u>Directions</u> and Total Time: approx. 20 minutes

Chop the pancetta and fry in a skillet over medium heat for 5 minutes until crispy. Set aside to cool. Mix spinach, lettuce, egg, and spring onion in a bowl. Whisk the vinaigrette ingredients in another bowl. Pour the dressing over, toss to combine. Top with avocado and pancetta. Serve immediately

Per serving: Cal 547; Fat 51g; Net Carbs 4g; Protein 12g

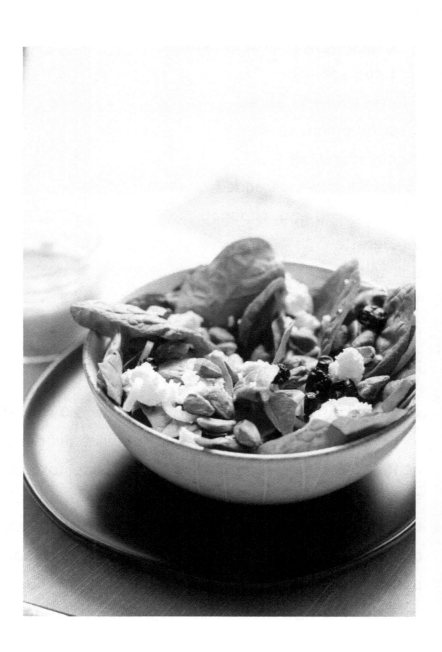

Mediterranean Artichoke Salad

Ingredients for 2 servings

6 baby artichoke hearts, halved

½ lemon, juiced

½ red onion, sliced

¼ cup cherry peppers, halved

¼ cup pitted olives, sliced

¼ cup olive oil

¼ tsp lemon zest

2 tsp balsamic vinegar

1 tbsp chopped dill

Salt and black pepper to taste

1 tbsp capers

Directions and Total Time: approx. 30 minutes

Bring a pot of salted water to a boil. Add in the artichokes. Lower the heat and let simmer for 20 minutes until tender. Drain and place the artichokes in a bowl to cool.

Add in the rest of the ingredients, except for the olives; toss to combine well. Top with the olives and serve.

Per serving: Cal 464; Fat 32g; Net Carbs 9.5g; Protein 13g

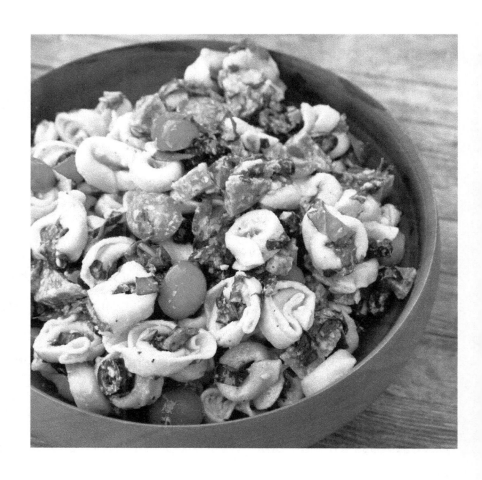

Arugula & Watercress Turkey Salad

Ingredients for 4 servings

1 tbsp xylitol

1 red onion, chopped

2 tbsp lime juice

3 tbsp olive oil

1 ¾ cups raspberries

1 tbsp Dijon mustard

Salt and black pepper, to taste

1 cup arugula

1 cup watercress

½ lb turkey breasts, boneless

4 oz goat cheese, crumbled

½ cup walnut halves

Directions and Total Time: approx. 25 minutes

Start with the dressing: In a blender, combine xylitol, lime juice, 1 cup raspberries, pepper, mustard, ¼ cup water, onion, olive oil, and salt and pulse until smooth. Strain this into a bowl and set aside.

Heat a pan over medium heat and grease lightly with cooking spray. Coat the turkey with salt and black pepper and cut in half. Place skin side down into the pan. Cook for 8 minutes, flipping to the other side and cooking for 5 minutes. Place arugula and watercress in a salad platter, scatter with the remaining raspberries, walnut halves, and goat cheese. Slice the turkey, put over the salad, and top with raspberries dressing to serve.

Per serving: Cal 511; Fat 35g; Net Carbs 7.5g; Protein 37g

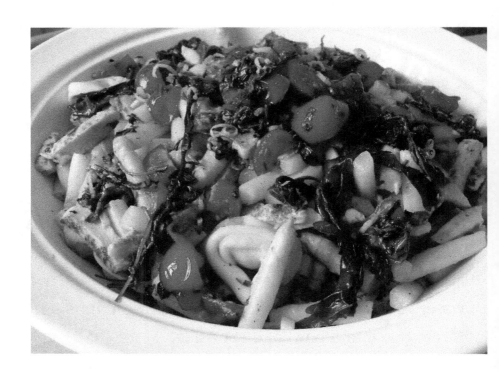

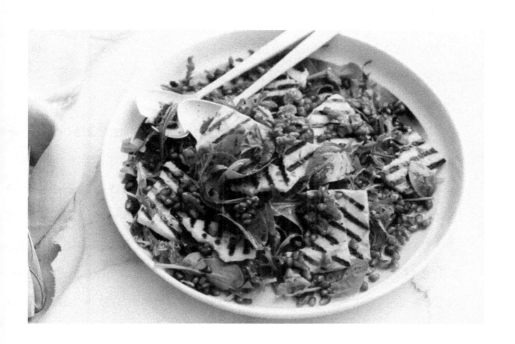

Spinach Salad with Goat Cheese & Nuts

Ingredients for 2 servings

2 cups spinach

½ cup pine nuts

1 cup hard goat cheese, grated

2 tbsp white wine vinegar

2 tbsp extra virgin olive oil

Salt and black pepper, to taste

Directions and Total Time: approx. 20 min + cooling time

Preheat oven to 390 F. Place the grated goat cheese in two circles on two parchment paper pieces. Place in the oven and bake for 10 minutes. Find two same bowls, place them upside down, and carefully put the parchment paper on top to give the cheese a bowl-like shape. Let cool that way for 15 minutes. Divide spinach among the bowls, sprinkle with salt and pepper, and drizzle with vinegar and olive oil. Top with pine nuts to serve.

Per serving: Cal 410; Fat 32g; Net Carbs 3.4g; Protein 27g

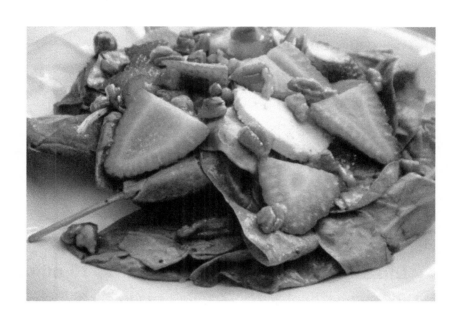

Thai-Style Prawn Salad

Ingredients for 2 servings

2 cups watercress

1 green onion, sliced

½ lb prawns, cooked

1 avocado, sliced

1 Thai chili pepper, sliced

1 tomato, sliced

1 tbsp cilantro, chopped

¼ tsp sesame seeds

1 tbsp lemon juice

2 tsp liquid stevia

½ tsp fish sauce

1 tbsp sesame oil

Directions and Total Time: approx. 20 minutes

In a bowl, whisk the stevia, sesame oil, fish sauce, and lemon juice. Add the prawns and toss to coat. Refrigerate covered for 10 minutes. Combine watercress, avocado, tomato, Thai chili pepper, and green onion on a serving platter. Top with prawns and drizzle the marinade over. Sprinkle with sesame seeds and cilantro and serve.

Per serving: Cal 420; Fat 29g; Net Carbs 1.8g; Protein 29g

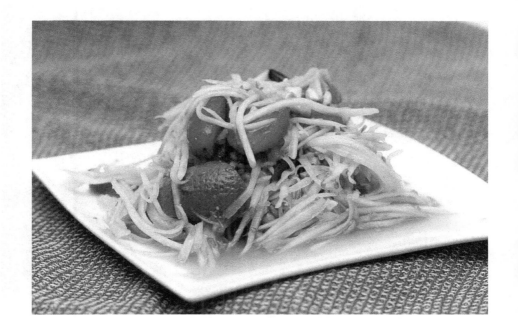

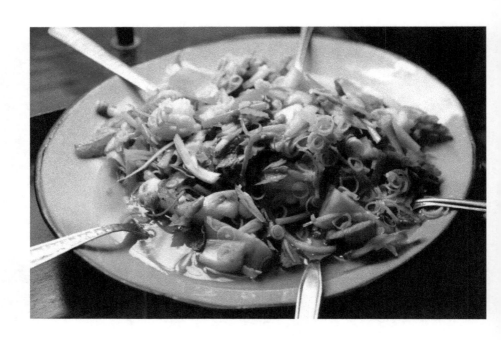

Modern Greek Salad with Avocado

<u>Ingredients</u> for 2 servings

1 red bell pepper, roasted and sliced

2 tomatoes, sliced

1 avocado, sliced

6 kalamata olives

¼ lb feta cheese, sliced

1 tbsp vinegar

1 tbsp olive oil

1 tbsp parsley, chopped

<u>Directions</u> and Total Time: approx. 10 minutes

Arrange the tomato slices on a serving platter and place the avocado slices in the middle. Place the olives and bell pepper around the avocado slices and drop pieces of feta on the platter. Drizzle with olive oil and vinegar and sprinkle with parsley to serve.

Per serving: Cal 411; Fat 35g; Net Carbs 5.2g; Protein 13g

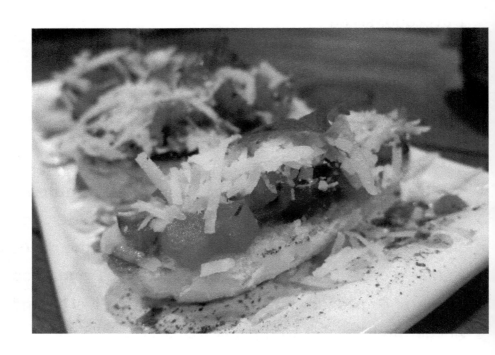

Seared Rump Steak Salad

Ingredients for 2 servings

1 cup green beans, steamed and sliced

½ lb rump steak

3 green onions, sliced

3 tomatoes, sliced

1 avocado, sliced

2 cups Romaine lettuce, torn

2 tsp yellow mustard

Salt and black pepper to taste

3 tbsp extra virgin olive oil

1 tbsp balsamic vinegar

Directions and Total Time: approx. 20 minutes

In a bowl, mix the mustard, salt, black pepper, balsamic vinegar, and extra virgin olive oil. Set aside.

Preheat a grill pan over high heat while you season the meat with salt and pepper. Place the steak in the pan and brown for 4 minutes per side. Remove to a chopping board and let it sit for 4 minutes before slicing.

In a salad bowl, add the green onions, tomatoes, green beans, lettuce, and steak slices. Drizzle the dressing over and toss to coat. Top with avocado slices and serve.

Per serving: Cal 611; Fat 45g; Net Carbs 6.4g; Protein 33g

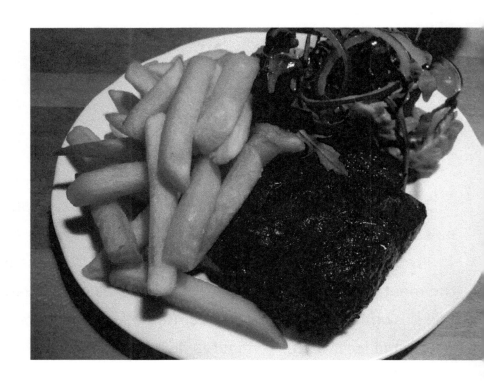

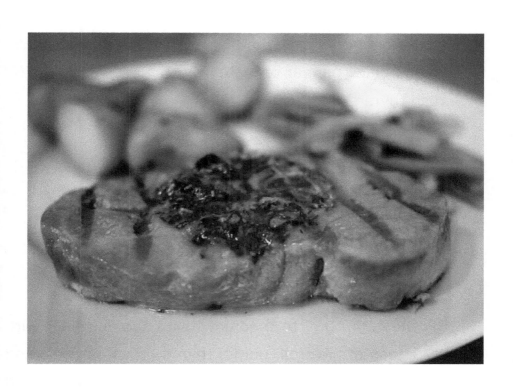

Cheesy Beef Salad

Ingredients for 4 servings

½ lb beef rump steak, cut into strips

1 tsp cumin

3 tbsp olive oil

Salt and black pepper to taste

1 tbsp thyme

1 garlic clove, minced

½ cup ricotta, crumbled

½ cup pecans, toasted

2 cups baby spinach

1 ½ tbsp lemon juice

¼ cup fresh mint, chopped

Directions and Total Time: approx. 15 minutes

Preheat the grill to medium heat. Rub the beef with salt, 1 tbsp of olive oil, garlic, thyme, black pepper, and cumin. Place on the preheated grill and cook for 10 minutes, flipping once.

Sprinkle the pecans on a dry pan over medium heat and cook for 2-3 minutes, shaking frequently. Remove the grilled beef to a cutting board, leave to cool, and slice into strips. In a salad bowl, combine baby spinach with mint, remaining olive oil, salt, lemon juice, ricotta, and pecans, and toss well to coat. Top with the beef slices.

Per serving: Cal 437; Fat 42g; Net Carbs 4.2g; Protein 16g

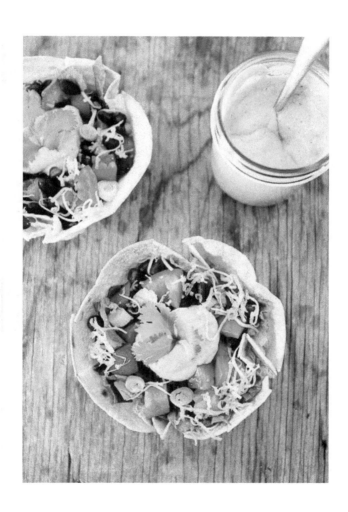

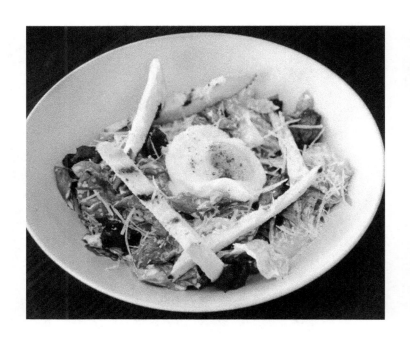

Pickled Pepper Salad with Grilled Steak

Ingredients for 2 servings

½ cup feta cheese, crumbled

1 lb skirt steak, sliced

Salt and black pepper to taste

1 tsp olive oil

1 cup lettuce salad

1 cup arugula

3 pickled peppers, chopped

2 tbsp red wine vinegar

Directions and Total Time: approx. 15 minutes

Preheat grill to high heat. Season the steak slices with salt and black pepper and drizzle with olive oil. Grill the steaks on each side to the desired doneness, about 5-6 minutes. Remove to a bowl, cover, and leave to rest while you make the salad. Mix the lettuce salad and arugula, pickled peppers, and vinegar in a salad bowl. Add the beef and sprinkle with feta cheese.

Per serving: Cal 633; Fat 34g; Net Carbs 4.7g; Protein 72g

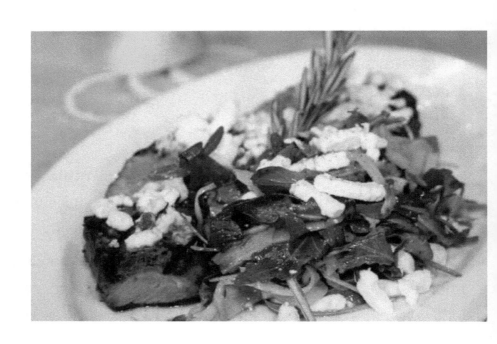

Parma Ham & Egg Salad

Ingredients for 4 servings

8 eggs

1/3 cup mayonnaise

1 tbsp minced onion

½ tsp mustard

1 ½ tsp lime juice

Salt and black pepper, to taste

10 lettuce leaves

4 Parma ham slices

Directions and Total Time: approx. 20 minutes

Boil the eggs for 10 minutes in a pot filled with salted water. Remove and run under cold water. Then peel and chop. Transfer to a mixing bowl together with the mayonnaise, mustard, black pepper, lime juice, onion, and salt. Top with lettuce leaves and ham slices to serve.

Per serving: Cal 723; Fat 53g; Net Carbs 5.6g; Protein 47g

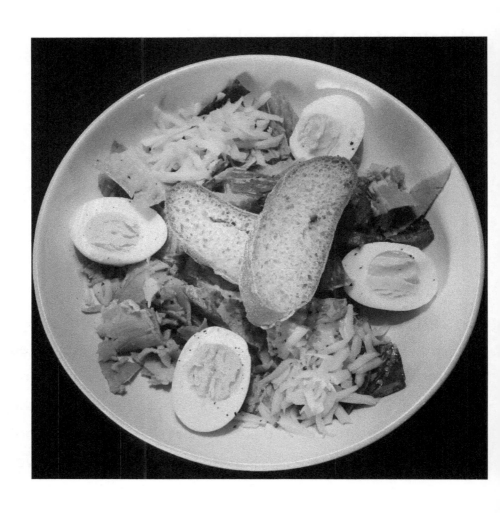

Chicken Salad with Gorgonzola Cheese

Ingredients for 2 servings

½ cup gorgonzola cheese, crumbled

1 chicken breast, boneless, skinless, flattened

Salt and black pepper to taste

1 tbsp garlic powder

2 tsp olive oil

1 cup arugula

1 tbsp red wine vinegar

Directions and Total Time: approx. 15 minutes

Rub the chicken with salt, black pepper, and garlic powder. Heat half of the olive oil in a pan over medium heat and fry the chicken for 4 minutes on both sides or until golden brown. Remove to a cutting board and let cool before slicing.

Toss the arugula with vinegar and the remaining olive oil; share the salads onto plates. Arrange the chicken slices on top and sprinkle with gorgonzola cheese.

Per serving: Cal 291; Fat 24g; Net Carbs 3.5g; Protein 12g

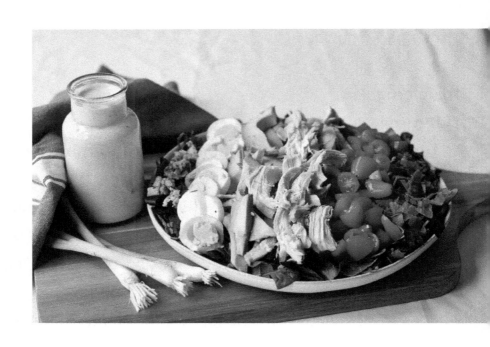

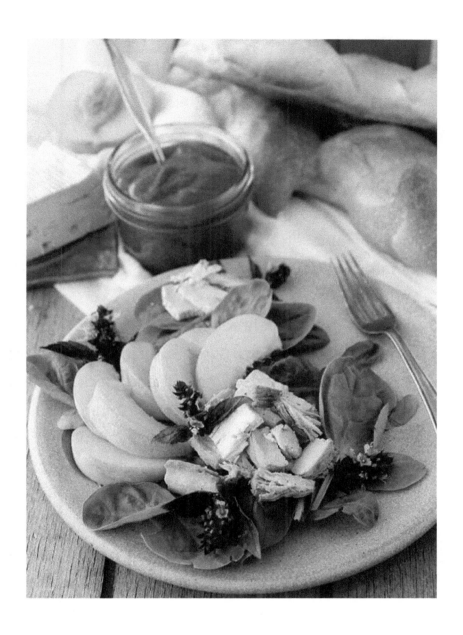

Cheddar & Turkey Meatball Salad

Ingredients for 4 servings

3 tbsp olive oil

1 tbsp lemon juice

1 lb ground turkey

Salt and black pepper to taste

1 head romaine lettuce, torn

2 tomatoes, sliced

¼ red onion, sliced

3 oz yellow cheddar, shredde d

Directions and Total Time: approx. 30 minutes

Mix the ground turkey with salt and black pepper and shape into meatballs. Refrigerate for 10 minutes.

Heat half of the olive oil in a pan over medium heat. Fry the meatballs on all sides for 10 minutes until browned and cooked within. Transfer to a wire rack to drain oil. Mix the lettuce, tomatoes, and red onion in a salad bowl, season with the remaining olive oil, salt, lemon juice, and pepper. Toss and add the meatballs on top. Scatter the cheese over the salad and serve.

Per serving: Cal 312; Fat 22g; Net Carbs 1.9g; Protein 19g

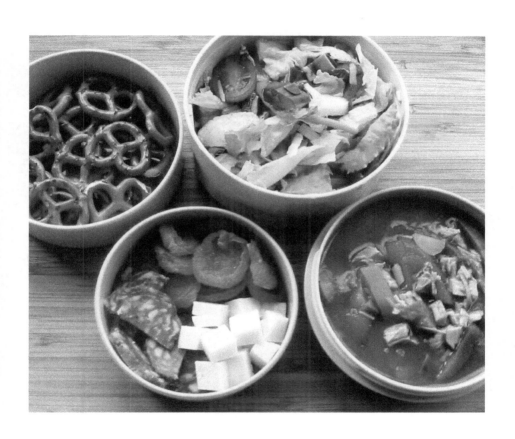

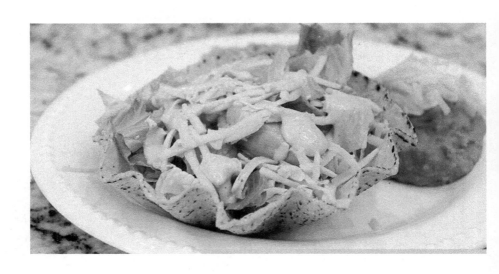